Dedicated to Nile and Eden.
You are the wind beneath my wings.

I almost died
That is for sure
For what I have
There is no man made cure.
Faith, hope, and standing on God's word
Is what I have to believe,
Anything else then I will be deceived.
What a huge task
To be entrusted with,
What a huge calling
To be faced with.
Death, I look you in your face
And I say no,
God is obviously not ready
for me to go.
Hair is falling out
Fingernails are black,
Eyebrows disappearing
My focus is whack.
Mommy, wife, friend daughter, employee,
Counselor, financial planner, travel coordinator,
Party planner, minister.
These are just some of the hats I wear
I have to take some hats off,
Do I dare?
There is one hat I need for sure,
The survivor hat

I must endure.
Gotta see my kids grow up
Go to college, start careers, get married,
have me some grand babies .
Gotta teach them how to eat,
how to stay healthy.
Gotta teach them grown up rights from wrongs
And that being wealthy is not
Having success,
Gotta teach them how to save and the
importance
Of paying off debts.
I almost died
That is for sure
For what I have
There is no man made cure.
Faith, hope, and standing on God's word
Is what I have to believe,
Anything else then I will be deceived.

INTRODUCTION

"Aweeeee!! I butchered myself!" This is my jerk reaction more times than I care to admit, when I look in the mirror after getting out of the shower. It's as if I am seeing myself for the first time. I do a silent scream. I have a moment where I ask why did I do it? I didn't have to go this extreme. Did I? Was this really necessary? And then those last fatal sad and depressing words, "who is gonna want you, with your scars and no boob stimulation whatsoever? You have mutilated yourself." It has been almost 6 years since my double mastectomy with reconstruction, and I still have this shocking trauma and view of myself. After about 1.5-3 minutes of that, I get myself together saying "whatever". "Whatever" has become like an empowering word. It's become my go to word when I feel like I am right on the edge about to fall. It's my saving grace. It's "whatever, I am still here. Whatever! My kids needed me. Whatever, it was not my time." It's the "whatever" that then removes my hands from uneven reconstructed barbie boobs and reaches for my toothbrush and toothpaste to start my day. Finally, it's the "whatever" that says "Thank G-d

For Big Boobs" because they are the same ripped up boobs that saved my very life.

Theologically Thinking

The enemy comes to distract.

BUT G-D!!

MY STORY

I was 39 when I was diagnosed with Stage III Breast Cancer. The cancer had spread to my lymph nodes. They removed 14 lymph nodes during surgery and found 4 in those. I was already dealing with life issues at the time with a marriage separation, and then a diagnosis like this should have rocked me in my boots. I can remember at one point not really knowing how to feel. My faith was being tested. My faith teaches me that "I am healed and that I can get through anything." I knew all the "faith" words to say but my reality was that I was just told that I was dying and that if I do some major things, I had a good chance of surviving.

I had two young daughters and did not have time to die. My daughters needed me. I couldn't cause that kind of pain on my daughters. I thought of everyone but myself. Ultimately, it was my faith that helped me and continues to provide medicine to my soul. I also believe as it goes to my soul that it also effects my body and can fight off illness. I believe that my faith and the hope in that the double mastectomy, chemo, radiation and hormonal therapy would work. Most importantly my faith and hope was in G-d that G-d knows best. I had to go to a higher faith that said, if it's my time, it's my time, and I'm okay with that and everyone will be okay in time as well. There are measures of faith that we grab on to when needed. I also, pulled on the faith of my family and friends who constantly poured words of strength and love into me.

I recall the time at my Pink Party, prior to my surgery, that I read words on some house shoes that were given as a gift. The house shoes read "Believe in a cure". It was that moment that I fully realized that I had something that had no cure. So, if there was no cure, that I could die? My best friend caught me reading it
and saw me drifting off and she immediately said "b$%#@, keep it moving!" Those words I will never forget. Her words said that we don't care what man says, we have faith in the Greatest Physician. You will be okay.

When I think of faith, hope and illness, I am reminded of the woman in the Bible, in Matthew Chapter 9 who had an issue of blood and who had radical faith! She had been hemorrhaging for 12 years. She was rendered legally uncleaned. She heard that the Messiah, Jesus, was coming to town and made a quality decision that day that if she even just touched the hem (like a hanging thread) of his clothing, that she could be healed. There were many following Jesus and the Disciples. Through the multitude of people she managed to tough the hem of Jesus' garment. "But Jesus turned him about, and when he saw her, he said, Daughter, be of good comfort; thy faith hath made thee whole. And the woman was made whole from that hour." (Matthew 9:22, KJV) That's radical faith! Her radical faith gave her medicine to her bleeding body instantly! She didn't have to wait. She didn't have to make an appointment. She was healed the very moment her faith touched Jesus. Faith is like medicine to the soul and can be medicine to the body too. The dis- ease in her body was gone. Whatever caused the dis-eased was possibly healed through her faith which ultimately healed her body! Dis-ease, I believe stems from environmental issues mostly. Even if genetic, I ask, how did the first person get it? This is a great example of how faith activated out of the hope of suffering no more, got the desired results instantaneously. Radical faith.

As a Minister, and as a Breast Cancer Survivor, I am even thankful for the radical faith of some scientists and doctors. Medicine is helping people to stay alive and helping people to experience more life. Every time we take a pill, it is in faith. We are believing that the pill will do what we are told it will do. We have faith that the doctor has faith in knowing what to tell us. We have faith that we will be given more opportunities to hopefully tell others how we survived.

With so much pain and suffering and traumatic situations, one wonders why some make it and some don't. This is a question I often wonder about myself. I wasn't even sick when I got my diagnosis. I did not feel a lump or anything weird going on. However, I wanted a breast reduction. It is something I had thought about for a while as my breasts were larger than I cared for them to be and I had back pain. I had gotten approved in 2010 by my insurance, but I chickened out. Then the following year, while my approval was still good, I decided to go for it. I found a Plastic Surgeon and we proceeded with the process. In doing so, I had to get a mammogram. That is when my entire life changed. From the mammogram came an ultrasound and biopsies and finally a diagnosis of Breast Cancer. Realizing that I had something that there was no cure for and that I could die absolutely changed the very core of my being. I often wonder why did my thoughts go towards my breast? Why was my life spared? My Primary Care Physician says "Be Thankful for big boobs", which shaped the title of this book. If I did not have big boobs, it is a good chance I would not be have written this book. I may not have seen my oldest daughter graduate from high school or my youngest grow "boobs" of her own. The only answer I have for being allowed to stay here on earth is that there is more work for me to do. There are lives for me to touch. There is something about my life that has to remain here.

"Thank G-d For Big Boobs!"

REFLECTION:
ARE THEY TALKING TO ME?

"Time spent in self-reflection is never wasted- it is an intimate date with yourself."
- Paul TP Wong

Day 4 AFTER DIAGNOSIS

Well, I woke up this morning! I am very thankful to all of my loved ones for all your support. I want to thank everyone in advance for all of the future support/prayers they will be providing as well. I didn't pinch myself today. I am coming to terms with the diagnosis. Don't get me wrong. I am not receiving sickness and just preparing to receive whatever G-d is doing and/or preparing me for. Who knows? Maybe I am being pushed towards purpose. After all, in the entire year of 2010 that was my prayer. To be in purpose on purpose. To walk in purpose on purpose. Now, I did not have ANY of this in mind. Trust me when I say that.

This all started with me wanting to get a breast reduction. My back has been hurting since 2004 in combination with issues with my Iliotibial band. This would cause me pain and the incapability of walking for long periods of time.

Anyway, the surgery was approved and was just weeks away from it. I had to get a mammogram and WHAM! My life is changed. We don't know yet if it has spread to my other breast yet. I get the MRI tomorrow. So send a prayer up, cross your fingers, and/or send positive energy my way. Whatever it is you do. But you know what I say; let's let G-d's will be done. I believe that everything will work out just as it should. I do believe my breasts will definitely be reduced. LOL! I said I wanted them reduced not gone! LOL! I was watching a part in a movie today where the young lady put on this beautiful panty and bra set for her husband and she stood there looking all fancy for him. He played like he was sleep. I cried. I was thinking about how I may have no breasts to fill up a pretty bra like hers. But then I wiped my tears and remembered implants. Then I remembered strapless tops and dresses that I may not even need a bra for!!! Woo hoo!! Ya see, that is not currently even an OPTION!! I would have so many more options. Then I may lose some weight with the chemo! This is not looking so bad after all! Now, if I can focus on that and not the fighting for my life and pain of it all, I'll be okay. This is day 4 of my diagnosis.

Day 5

MRI today. Don't feel much like writing today. Have a blessed day.

Day 8

Well guys, I am still waiting on the results of the MRI, the remaining biopsy results and genetics testing. I sit patiently waiting on the phone to ring. Church was good. I went to my family's church yesterday. The girl Amber from the TV show Sunday's Best visited and sang her hiney off! I mean everyone was on their feet with arms lifted. She sang a song called Total Praise. Loved it!! The Pastor, who is also my cousin, preached and I felt like he was talking directly to me. He preached from John 9 versus 1-5. The part that got me was verse 3. This scripture is talking about a man who was born blind.

"Neither this man nor his parents sinned," said Jesus, "but this happened so that the works of G-d might be displayed in him....."

I could not help but think about me and my lil situation. Not so little, but hey, I'm gonna call it a "lil situation" today. Wow! Did you hear what that scripture said, "so that the works of G-d might be displayed in ME". I'm changing the last word from "him" to "me".   I understand that G-d will never give me more than I can handle. I will just continue to trust him. No. His ways are not our way. Not at all. But He is doing something behind the scenes and only he holds the blueprint. It may not feel good, it may not be necessarily a happy time. But I will say to G-d be the glory.

I may not feel up to saying much in a couple of weeks, so I'll say it out loud now. To G-d be the Glory! I'm still trusting you Lord! I really hope this is pushing me towards purpose even more clearly, cuz I'm tired of trying to figure it all out.

Day 10- REALLY?

"CALM MIND BRINGS INNER STRENGTH AND
SELF-CONFIDENCE, SO THATS VERY IMPORTANT
FOR GOOD HEALTH."
-DALAI LAMA

Ok...so yesterday I had a "moment". I had to schedule my ultrasound and then the Scheduler said "we will go ahead and schedule your biopsy right after the ultrasound just in case anything looks like we need more information." ANOTHER BIOPSY? Oh excuse me...MAYBE 2 because they need to look at 1 in my left boob AND another one in my right.

Sooooooooooooooo. I left work and went down the street to my weekly work Bible study.....calmed down....remembered that I am a strong woman with G-d holding my hands.....and eventually went back to work. This journey is just starting y'all. It is not easy, I keep saying it could be worst. I will get through it. We will get through this.

Day 11- Lil "c" ain't got nothin on Big J!

"We may encounter many defeats but we must not be defeated."
- Dr. Maya Angelou

As I was driving in I was thinking, cancer does not seem the same to me now. I guess cuz the docs say I have it. OK. I'll admit, I think they are talking to me. LOL However, I will not give it power. It will always be cancer with a little "c" for me. I was just thinking of that old saying, "what doesn't kill you will make you stronger". It's just one of those things. It's just a challenge. It's my challenge. Apparently I can handle it. My G-d may not have created this lil "c " but He is allowing it to go on. Perhaps it is my testimony. Maybe even my platform. The timing of it all sucks. But I will survive and look back and give a sigh of relief. Or maybe o my next ultrasound it will be all gone!!!!

When I get down and I ask one of my BFFs to remind me of who I am , and my Hydrack BFF says: "You are the BOMB! Gorgeous! Talented! Virtuous! Our valedictorian! Our 1st runner up in talent Ms. Teen! Our almost board member!

Dynamic mother! Writer! Ideator! Our play headliner! Girl...hush yo mouth you are the BOMB!!" Hee Hee! Love her! All of my BFFs and friends and family are amazing!

When you are going through something, surround yourself with people who understand you and love you!!

"Life and death is in the power of the tongue!" I speak LIFE!!
I've got the power!!!

I can do it !

I am walking in healing!!

Day 14- Just wanting to know

**"Do the best you can until you know better.
Then when you know better,
do better."
- Dr. Maya Angelou**

Well. It's been 2 weeks since the doctors been talking all this stuff. I am waiting for my surgeon to call me again so we can go over some details of the surgery. I just want to know if I need to cut them all off or if it looks like I can save a little. My main thing is that I don't want it coming back....so I am mentally preparing myself for whatever, but I just want to know..."whatever". I want to know radiation or chemo or both. I want to know if I am moving towards Stage 2 with these new findings. I just want to know. I NEED to know.

I ......never mind…

Day 15, I guess. I Think They are Talking to Me

Well, went to my plastic surgeon today to go over options. Looked at lots and lots of previous patients who had lil breasts. Y'all, it's crazy but I am not feeling radiation. It totally shrinks your breast and then possibly shifts your nipple sideways or under. So if I do a lumpectomy and reduction, the boob may still be out of whack after radiation. As crazy as it is sounding, a mastectomy is not sounding bad.....and most importantly I don't want "lil c" coming back to haunt me. I would do chemo w/ no radiation if I do the mastectomy. This is all so much. I don't think I want to go to another doctor's appointment alone. I'm a big girl but it's too much information and I am just tired.
So:
Lumpectomy and radiation (chemo maybe): Keep my own breast but all kind of asymmetry- not mentioning the redness, swelling and burning.

Mastectomy: Lose your breasts completely, get an expander; may need skin from back; implant; chemo; more symmetry .

(Keep in mind, studies show that lumpectomy w/ radiation works as well as mastectomy w/ chemo in many cases.)

Waiting on genetic testing and results from the ultrasound and possible additional biopsy or 2, I am doing on Friday. May not have a choice of procedure when these things come back.

As of today, surgery is scheduled for October 6th.

Day 16- I think

Well, it's a new day. Just spoke with the Oncologist's office. I'll probably meet with them towards the end of October. I am still amazed that I have this lil cancer (oxymoron I know), and that it is something that if i don't treat it can spread and my life could end. That does not scare me for me, but it concerns me for my children and my family. Nevertheless, it will be treated, it will go away. And that's that!!

Today, I am coming to terms with possibly having a mastectomy. Not because I am not optimistic, but simply because I don't want it to come back. I saw all those radiation pictures and the possibility of additional future surgeries is just not appealing, unless I want to walk around lop sided. Ummm. No. I have never been a vain person, but I don't know anyone who would want one breast longer than the other one. I am 39 years old. Full of life and I do like to look nice. I like to look good, jazzy and rock ethnic styles. Bottom line, I want even boobs if I am going to have them.

Anyway. today I am just wrapping my mind around cutting off my boobs and getting implants.

Dancing like there was no tomorrow!

"Life isn't about waiting for the storm to pass...It's learning to dance in the rain."
-Anonymous

Ok, so we had our 25th Company Anniversary at work. It was at the City Museum. There was food, scavenger hunt games, adult beverages, music and a dance floor! And y'all!!! I danced like there was no tomorrow! lol I mean, normally I will dance a little, keep it reserved, cute and fun. But last night! We danced! I danced! We had a great time, my coworkers and I danced. I mean, we just felt the music. I did a little lyrical, a little ballet, electric slide, cha cha slide, wobble wobble, you name it! I did the snake and the smurf! Ole school! I played a little pee a boo with this pole!! It was a wide pole so no pole dancing people. REALLY?!! LOL! It was so awesome!!! I just decided to let my hair down and dance and be funny and silly and just have a great time!!! Luckily!! I had other folks around me doing the same thing!!! This was the bunch who stayed while "others" left. We were the second shift and the party got even better!! We made song requests and pulled folks on the dance floor. Shout out to S who danced all night!!! Shout out to "L" who slid down the slide with me for GP!!! Shout out to the DJ who kept it moving with all styles of music.

I had the best time with folk I work with, but barely really know. But last night on the dance floor we were all friends. Last night for a moment, I forgot I had cancer. It was a great time!

Dance

                    Dance

Dance

Day 21- Amazing Day

Well...so Friday I went for my Ultrasound and chickened out on the biopsy. The Radiologist wanted to do 2 biopsies...1 for the left and the 2nd thing they see on the right. I think he thinks the right one maybe another cancer but the left looks like more of a fibroid. If I get a bilateral mastectomy, I couldn't remember why the biopsy would be necessary on the left. Well, my doctor reminded me later on. She needs to know whether some lymph nodes need t be removed on that side as well. Nevertheless, her office called me bright and early this morning to get that scheduled. Still waiting on the day and time. But it will be this week I am sure.

Ok...so I had a lovely surprise. I went to my high school's all alumni picnic a couple of months ago and met two wonderful people who took me under their wing like their little sister. See, no one from the class of 1990 was really there and I felt so out of place. Well, one of the ladies and I have facebooked and we spoke last night. Guess what?! She is a breast cancer survivor!!! G-d never ceases to AMAZE me. I believe G-d definitely put her in my life for this appointed time. We talked for hours during the Falcons vs

Philly game last night. She is awesome. I look forward to her coming to my Pink Party Brunch on Sunday! Not to mention that 2 of my BFFs (that I know of) are flying in!

Did I say how much I love my daughters? They are so lovely and special. So unique and amazing! I thank G-d for putting them in my life. They are my motivation for living.

ANOTHER DAY

"Wisdom is nothing more than healed pain."
Anonymous

Well...just got back from the biopsy for my other breast. Sting sting, numb numb, click click click and it's done. But you have to turn your head away from looking at the huge device (needle) that is used. Gosh! I think I may be able to climb a mountain when everything is said and done!

I am actually a little sore. I have an ice pack on but I will admit there is a lil discomfort. But it's all okay.

Results back on Thursday. Still waiting on the genetics testing results.

I love you all!!

They ARE Talking To Me- Out of Body Experience

"The comeback is always stronger than the setback."
- Anonymous

OK, so they are talking to me. It is what it is. I had the biopsy in the left breast yesterday. Went well, if there is a such thing. I should have the results my tomorrow. This is truly an out of body experience. Those who are closest to me know all that I am dealing with and it's just a bit much. I will say, when I come out of this, I will be better and stronger than ever. I am going to live and enjoy this life. The fact that I have realized that I have a disease that if I don't treat it, will kill my physical body, is an eye opener. I could literally be dead within a matter of years. That is absolutely crazy! Thank G-d for medicine and research!! I want to live. I choose life. If it means losing my breasts. I choose life! If losing my breasts will give me another 40 years to experience watching my daughters grow into women and maybe even wives and moms too. I choose life!

They are talking to me and I choose life!

They must be Talking to me!! PINK PARTY!!

October 4th

SO WHAT! They Are Talking To Me

"What doesn't kill me, makes me stronger. So if you plan to hurt me, make sure you kill me or I'll be coming back for you."
-iliketoquote.com

Ok so what. They are talking to me. Surgery is in 2 days and I know I have not blogged in a while.

Gotta lot on my mind and really don't feel like saying much.

I am trusting G-d!!!

Healing- Post Surgery

"Learning is a gift. Even when pain is your teacher."
-Dr. Maya Angelou

I am healing 1 day at a time. Pain is an understatement at times....discomfort may even be better. BUT I am here and I am thankful for life.

I have not felt like typing, so I have not been on here in some days. I can't wait for the day that I just feel good again physically. The pain has kept me from dealing with the psychological things yet. But that's okay. G-d is working everything out. G-d is my healer and I just love G-d. G-d sent me friends and family to be here for me. I am so thankful.

8 days post surgery

OUCH!! The Lord is my healer and I thank G-d for drugs to get through the excruciating pain. I thank G-d for family and friends.

Got some saline put in the expanders, so it's tighter in addition to the pain. It will be okay and I will get through it.. We will get through it. Purpose is standing ahead of me.

Keeping it Real

I trust G-d. I been trusting G-d far beyond this cancer stuff. I just trust even more. I have to give up so much humanly control that it is very humbling. Fighting depression is normal. And crying is a daily routine. Oftentimes, tears of joy from the acts of love that I am receiving. My sister bathed me yesterday. I just sat there and cried just from that action alone. I am the oldest and I feel sad that my loved ones are having to do these things for me. I am just not used to receiving so much. I am so moved and touched.

I recognize that I need to over load myself on healing songs and scriptures as my mind gets attacked with thoughts of there not being a cure. I am concerned that because I am naturally optimistic and positive that I could slip up and wind up with a shorter life span than I envision. I remind myself that Jesus took this cancer ahead of time so that I can be cured of it. I am already healed. I must be reminded. I must make sure that I believe this without a shadow of a doubt.

Just thankful for my friends and family!

Thursday and Friday

"When you come out of the storm you won't be the same person that walked in. That's what the storm is all about."
-Haruki Murakami

Ok...so...Thursday I have the Plastic Surgeon appointment in the AM and the Radiation appointment in the PM.

Friday- Chemo appt.

Wooo Hooo!! Bring it on!!! Sometimes you gotta go through the storm to get to your purpose.
I trust you G-d! Jehovah Rapha.

"We want to get to the resurrection without the crucifixion!" I heard that recently from someone and thought I'd share.

MORE Healing

"Honest feelings and bad timing make the most painful combination."
-www.livelifehappy.com

I am healing 1 day at a time. Pain is an understatement at times....discomfort may even be better. BUT I am here and I am thankful for life.

I have not felt like typing, so I have not been writing in some days. I can't wait for the day that I just feel good again physically. The pain has kept me from dealing with the psychological things yet. But that's okay.

G-d is working everything out.
G-d is my healer and I just love G-d.
G-d sent me friends and family to be here for me.
I am so thankful.

Blessed. People Care.

I am so blessed. So many wonderful people in my life. So many. I am brought to tears by so many acts of kindness. People taking care of me. People just stopping by to make sure I am ok. People taking me to doctors appointments. People calling asking if I need anything. People bringing food over. People sending flowers. People bringing me lunch. People sending me cards. People flying in and out of town to see me. People taking my kids to their sports games. People doing my kids' hair. People taking and picking my kids up from school. People taking my kids to Halloween parties. People taking my kids to the mall. And even today, people taking my youngest to see "Puss and Boots."

I am brought to tears. Who says that people don't care about people anymore? Well, I say I don't know what kind of people they know. But I know the kind of people who have a heart after G-d's. A giving spirit.

I am blessed.

And this will pass...

Okay....well chemotherapy starts tomorrow. I'm cool. I was more concerned about getting the chemo port than I am about the chemo. One more day closer to this stuff being over.

My tissue expanders are still uncomfortable. I don't recommend them personally. It's like 2 mini helmets being placed in your chest. I can't really sleep. I am off of pain meds just on a muscle relaxer. All I can say is help me Jesus. BUT it is better than what it was or I am just getting used to the pain. UGH!!

I have a little fluid in my right boob that should not be there. I am wearing cotton under the bra to hopefully help this problem. Be in prayer that infection does not come. That would be a bad thing. So that is not gonna happen!

Well, my lovely sister came over and cut my hair off. Took a picture. Not my best photo at all.

Here we go!
"If you even dream of beating me, you better
wake up and apologize."
- Muhammed Ali

Round 1

Well...I went ahead and got the chemo port which
I was struggling with, it ended up being a decent
process.
It was probably the best thing for me.

Just been sluggish. 1st day I was nauseated and
sluggish. These tissue expanders are the worst
of my problems. They are constantly painful. So I
am forced to take pain pills when I already have
so much crap in me.

My hair may start falling out in 2 weeks. I'm ready
if it does. Just ready to feel good again. These
expanders are the worst of it all. Well the cancer
is bad too.

Ice. Ice. Ice.
Tissue expanders!
Cannot recommend them!

Laughter

"I am not my hair. I am not my skin. I am the Soul that lives within."
-India Arie

I watched Bridesmaids, the movie, and laughed until I cried!! It was awesome. Best laugh in over 3 months!
I highly recommend it. I soooooooooooooooo needed that laugh! I mean it broke through a little depression and sadness. Laughter is great for the soul!

Let it shed let it shed let it sheddddddddddd!

Well......my hair is shedding. Yep. It's falling out. Scalp was feeling tingly , feels better now. I washed it with baby shampoo in the shower. Had a headache and eyes were red a few days this week. Yes indeed...chemo is kicking in. Do your thang chemo so I can get on with the rest of my life.

Crabby

"I hurt!"
-Jacqueline Knuckles McCall

Not a good day today. Cranky all day. Just don't feel good. Hair is shedding and boobs hurt.

I'm saying I am Healed!!

Well......ok....my hair is shedding. GOOD! That means the chemo is working. The chemo needs to kill off all the things that are not right. SO Good! Praise G-d! Praise Jehovah! Praise Yahweh!! Praise Go-d!!

I love the LORD, my healer, my provider. It is the G-d in me that will get me through this. Unfortunately my family and friends can not fix this. They can help me along the way and they have, and boy do I need it!! More than I can even vocalize.

My physical body is just catching up with my spiritual.

Staying calm

"Just do it."
-Nike

Ok so I was about to panic. My hair is falling out more and more. I see a spot that is about to be bald. Thank G-d I have a great supply of scarves and WIGS!! I happen to have about 4 or 5 wigs. Thanks to my friends and I had bought a couple this summer ironically, just because! It will be okay. It will be okay.

Oh wellllllllll

Good news. I don't have to see 1 of the docs anymore for 1 year!! Woo Hoo!! Making progress.

Now, I have a dilemma. Should I just go bald? Ya know very very low...I am already low but it's still coming out and I have a receding hair line like a guy.

Decisions

Chemo day today. I think I am just gonna go bald today.

Chemo

"Prayer is key to our heartbeat."
-Jacqueline Knuckles McCall

Ok. I am still here at chemo. Been at the hospital since before 2pm. It is now 7:32 pm. Lab work, doc appointment and then chemo. I think I am on my last batch. Like watching paint dry. Feel aight.

Tonight several of us getting chemo talked. It was nice. Pray for George 67 yrs...was in stage 4 cancer a few yrs ago.....went in remission and it's back now. I can tell he is a fighter and a friend of G-d.

Also, I met a young woman who has breast cancer. Diagnosed in July. Ended up with 2 different kind of cancers in 1 breast. It Metastasized and went to her liver. She had surgery . It sounds promising. I think she will be just fine. Why? Cuz we are Warriors!!!!

Mrs. Clean

I'm almost bald.

Round 2 was bad!

I'm bald and this 2nd round of chemo wiped me out. It is taking me about a week to get it together. Today is the first day I feel like talking to anyone.

Dec 13th

"Not that I speak in regard to need, for I have learned in whatever state I am, to be content: I know how to be abased, and I know how to abound. Everywhere and in all things I have learned both to be full and to be hungry, both to abound and to suffer need. I can do all things through Christ who strengthens me.
(Phil 4:11-13)

I think slowly but surely, I am getting to this contentment as I humbly appreciate life. Honestly, with this happening to me, I don't know what the future holds.

I don't know how long I have on earth. I think when you are faced with death, you have a new appreciation for life as you really understand better what it means that your life is in G-d's hands. I don't want to take for granted that I will be here for stuff even though I plan on it. I must prepare my daughters for life. I want them to be smart and not just book smart. Common sense smart will take one a long way. I want them to be strong and know that they can do whatever comes to mind. I want them to find passion for G-d, life and the universe around them. Travel.

Travel. Travel. See the world before creating their own family. Early 20s travel travel travel. Start a family late 20s early 30s. Get a good book education and life education before husbands and babies. Laugh!! Laugh! Laugh!! Eat healthy . Eat green. Juice. Be organized. It makes a difference. Don't procrastinate. Just do it! Pray first before all things. And I want them to know that I love them and will always be with them. I'll find a way!!! :)

3rd Round of chemo

I am half way done with chemo and 1 step closer to radiation.

Last Chemo was Feb 23rd!

I just finished chemo! Thank you Jesus! Next up radiation! 6 weeks Mon -Fri!

This has been a life changing event. I feel like I have to get to know myself again. I have to get used to what they call "the new normal". This has been a whirlwind. Diagnosis- surgery (losing body parts), pain, chemo, sick, and now radiation.

Vacation, vacation and vacation! Here I come.

Brand new outlook on life. Each day is precious. The sun even looks different.

Radiation is radiant!
Seriously?!
April 4th

Soooooooooooooo. I started radiation last week. I had to do a simulation first to get marked up and measured as to where the rays would go. I'll admit I was a bit traumatized. There were like 4 people marking , tattooing and taping me up all at the same time. I just laid there naked on top. Felt a little violated but why entertain those thoughts when nothing good will come from it.

Today will be day 7 of radiation

I know the routine. I leave work, I park, I go in and swipe my card, I go to the back and change from the waist up into the gown. I sit and wait for them to call my name. I tell them my name, dob, and tell them the area that is being treated. I go in the room, take my wig and shoes off. I lay down and then they position me. I ask them to cover my arms up because the room is freezing. They leave the room and then the machines begin to circle me. Then the rays come and I try to lay as still as possible for the next 15 minutes or so. It never fails that some itch pops up. So I try to think of everything but that itch.

This is my routine following a full day Monday, Tuesday, Wednesday, Thursday and Friday for 6 weeks.
People don't know how good they have it when healthy. Life is taken for granted. I will never take it for granted again. I want to live life happy and to the fullest. I am making life plans. Just got a few hurdles to leap. It also looks like I may have entered menopause (night sweats and flashes). The doctors don't know yet if it is temporary or permanent. Right! As if I needed anything else to deal with. But it is bad and funny! Not to complain, but I am already uncomfortable at night because of the expanders. Then to add sweating that awakes me, it's just not right. I sure hope I am learning whatever I am suppose to learn from all of this. I hope wisdom encircles me.

WHATEVER!

WHATEVER!

WHATEVER!

WHATEVER!

The BEGINNING- We made it!

Been a while.
So it's been a while since I wrote anything. I finished radiation successfully. I was red and blistered and in pain...but of course I SURVIVED!!!! I will have to catch you up on EVERYTHING soon.

Smooches!!

Guys, that's where my blogging ends and new life begins. Since then, I got those dreadful expanders out and implants in. What a relief. Recovery has been good overall. My memory is not my best, so I've learned to take notes when needed. One issue is lymphedema in my right arm and hand. During my breast surgery, 14 lymph nodes were removed. This has caused my lymphatic system on my right side not to operate as well, causing swelling. An arm sleeve and therapy helps. It did land me in the hospital for 3 days as I got cellulitis. That was painful. I never thought my arm could cause so much pain. It was like having a fever in your arm. It was literally hot, red and blotchy. During this incident, I discovered that I have 2 deep vein thrombosis blood clots in that arm. Currently, I am continuously dealing with swelling and have a hard time writing. But thank G-d for computers and texting! LOL!

Let's see what else. One thing I failed to mention during all of my treatment is the relationship between my THEN husband and I. We were actually separated when I received my diagnosis. Everything got postponed while I was treating, but we eventually divorced. Don't be sad for me. I am much happier now and he is too. I know that the cancer had a lot to do with my life rearranging. G-d works in mysterious ways. I believe that cancer was allowed in my life to push me forward in purpose. I currently relocated my daughters and I to North Carolina where I am finishing my Master of Divinity degree at Duke University, so I can be in full time ministry. My oldest daughter has begun college and my youngest is in high school. I also recently married an amazing man who loves all of me and my imperfections.

The Beginning

When told bad news you will deal with some of the following emotions:

Fear

Sadness

Disappointment

Anger

Regret

Defeat

Urgency

THIS IS NORMAL!

"Allow yourself to feel how you feel."
-Jacqueline Knuckles McCall

It's okay to cry. It's okay to feel grieved. You have experienced trauma. But just don't stay in that space. G-d has equipped us with everything we need to pull ourselves up out of the dump. That assistance can show up in a friend, a family member, a scripture, or any other way. Listen and let help come in. If you need time to feel the pain, communicate that so that others know you will come out, but you need time to process the information you are dealing with for now.

No matter what trial you are facing in your life, it is up to you to make quality decisions. Make sound decisions. Find the blessing in that which you believe tried to take you out. For me, my boobs tried to take me out, but at the same time I say "Thank G-d for Big Boobs!" If you live to tell your story, there is a testimony to be told. Thank G-d for that thorn in your side and see how you have grown or have the potential to grow from that thing. See how your relationship with G-d is renewed or grows. There is no time like the present time to get a new lease on life. There is no time like the present to reinvent yourself or make an improved version of yourself. Find purpose in the pain. When you find purpose in the pain, you'll find peace, and you'll feel better overall. No one said life would be easy. No one also said that we'd be exempt from problems. But we can control our reaction and can choose to see the glass full instead of half empty.

Lessons Learned (no particular order)

1. Don't sweat the small stuff
2. It's okay to be dependent on others
3. Focus on what G-d is saying to you
4. See G-d with a new lens
5. My beauty is not just based on my outward appearance
6. I am still desired and attractive
7. We must serve each other
8. My life is not my own
9. Teach our children things we did not know
10. I'm a better steward of my body
11. I am stronger than I know

Daily Tips

1. Be true to your feelings
2. Set boundaries that work for you
3. Be honest to others about how you feel
4. Don't be afraid to ask for help
5. Create a plan for family living during this time
6. Call on your village in advANCE to help with grocery shopping and needs
7. Create a mantra for yourself

Mantra Ideas (choose 3 or 4 and say daily until you believe them.)

I walk in love.
I walk in healing.
I walk in forgiveness.
I walk in strength.
I walk in calm.
I walk in grace,
I walk in peace.
I walk in faith.
I walk in blessings.
I walk in miracles.
I walk in G-d.

Throw a party!

Dear Valued Reader,

I pray that my story has shed some insight on what life can be like once diagnosed with an illness. There are days filled with ebs and flows. However, with faith in G-d, the love and help of family, friends and doctors who genuinely are concerned, one is able to persevere. Keep the faith.

"THANK G-D FOR BIG BOOBS!"

Walking in continuous healing,
Jackie

Photo Credit: Eddie Holman IV

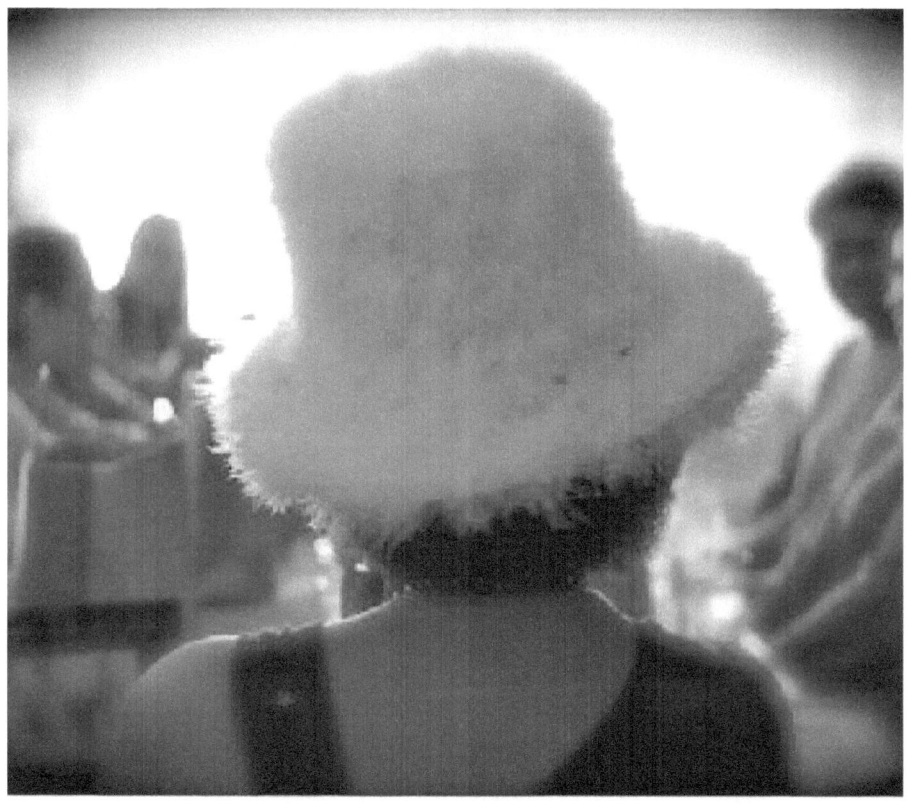

The ringing of the bell

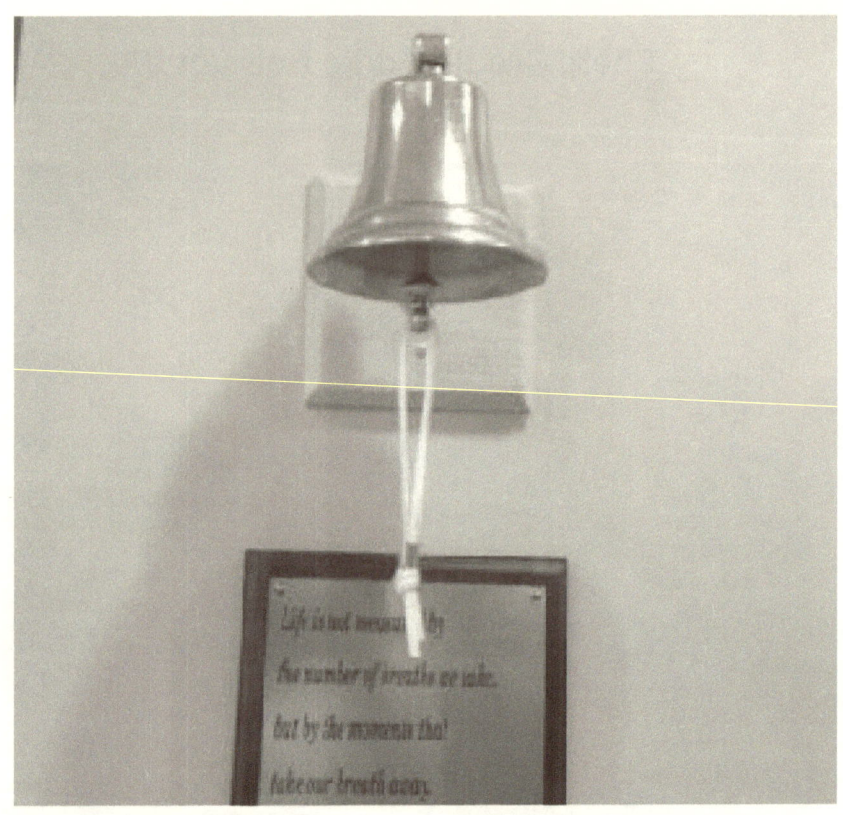

After the last chemotherapy treatment, we
ring this bell. I rang the heck out of it.
Everyone, everywhere could hear!
Then I cat walked right up out of there!

www.ingramcontent.com/pod-product-compliance
Lightning Source LLC
Chambersburg PA
CBHW031329290526
45784CB00014B/2451